The
Natural
Childbirth
Primer

By the Same Author

CHILDBIRTH WITHOUT FEAR

INTRODUCTION TO MOTHERHOOD

NO TIME FOR FEAR

The Natural Childbirth Primer

By GRANTLY DICK-READ
M.A., M.D. (Cantab.)

HARPER & ROW, PUBLISHERS
New York and Evanston

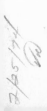

To Jess,

My dear wife and counselor

THE NATURAL CHILDBIRTH PRIMER

This book is published in England
under the title of *Antenatal Illustrated*

Library of Congress catalog card number: 56–6913

71 72 73 10 9

Contents

Illustrations

Preface

It is a privilege to write a preface to this small but important book. It is not often that an author is willing to state to others, "This is as much your work as mine, and without the part you played it could not have been written."

Men are at such a disadvantage when women's impressions of childbirth are discussed. There are so many reasons why I am dependent upon "the ladies" for, although by long years of observation the processes of natural childbirth became clear to me, I have remained unable to write of them as a personal achievement.

It is no secret that I have never had a baby, or taken a course of antenatal instruction. I have never denied this disability when indignant women have argued, "Has he ever had a baby? What does he know!" But those who have given me help to compile these pages are mothers who have borne babies naturally—I do thank them all for the willing way in which they posed for photographs of the various subjects illustrated.

For four years I practiced in Johannesburg, where this teaching became established, but my wife was shocked by the standard of antenatal preparation of the women in the "City of Gold." She started, therefore, on her own, a school where women could be trained and instructed for childbirth. She has no degrees or diplomas, but qualified in the school of experience and many years of close, companionable interest with me in my work.

Her first baby was born by an emergency Caesarean section

because of a severe illness, and her second was an entirely natural birth of a nine-pound boy.

Each woman who attended her classes became a subject of observation and research—several hundreds of them of many European nationalities. The object was to understand their difficulties and fears and to prepare their minds and bodies to have their babies naturally, at the same time to find the simplest way of achieving the best results. Her art of simplification of antenatal care spreads wherever natural childbirth is used and she was present at the deliveries of most of her pupils.

Her assistant continued to conduct the School of Instruction until the day before her own baby was born and that birth was a perfect example of the ideals my wife had for her pupils.

The illustrations are women in routine classes; they are not selected because of either ability or appearance and it is from hundreds like them that I, a mere man, learn so much and over the long years have been able to pass on a message of comfort to every civilized country in the world.

I am, therefore, sincerely grateful to those who have put into practice my teaching and procedures, but without my wife as an intermediary and counselor, I could not have gleaned the detailed knowledge of the strange activities in the mind of woman, that citadel whose secrets are not known to man.

G. D.-R.

Petersfield
December, 1955

The
Natural
Childbirth
Primer

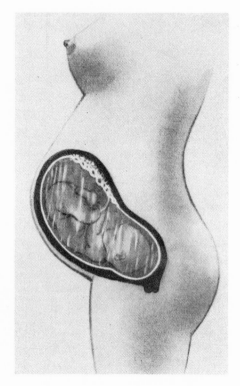

Fetus *in Utero* at Full Term

To Women Who Are Going
to Have Babies

OVER 95 per cent of women can have their babies safely and without unbearable discomfort. The birth of a child is a natural process and only the lack of preparation and understanding by both the patient and her attendant have brought it near to being a surgical operation. It is the most important event in a woman's life. The health and happiness of wives, husbands and families largely depend upon the care of women in childbirth.

It is the only job modern, civilized women are expected to be good at without any education or training; this is a mistake. There is reason to believe that even animals, in some way, hand down to their offspring the knowledge of how to bear their young and look after them when they are born. It may be called natural instinct, which is really being taught by some means we don't understand to do the right thing at the right moment.

All over the world today, women who are properly prepared for and looked after during labor experience a deep sense of satisfaction and joy in bearing children, and it is the right of every woman to be given that opportunity of learning how to make childbirth a happy event and not a hardship.

This small book cannot go into full details, but outlines briefly the four essentials which assist a normal, healthy woman to achieve her ambition of a natural birth and a healthy baby. In order of importance, women must be prepared by:

a. Education,
b. Correct breathing,
c. Relaxation, and finally
d. Exercises.

For those who want to learn more about these subjects, *Childbirth Without Fear,* Revised and Enlarged Edition, and my smaller book, *Introduction to Motherhood* (both published in the United States by Harper & Brothers), explain all aspects of pregnancy and childbirth. The more completely wives and husbands understand pregnancy and childbirth the easier it becomes for each of them to avoid anxiety and to find companionship in family life.

As far back as we know anything about the human race, having babies has been a necessary and natural part of living. But about one hundred years ago, chloroform and antiseptics (1865) were discovered. These wonderful boons to surgery made it both easier and safer to interfere with the normal and natural processes of childbirth, and the era of Meddlesome Midwifery commenced. It was accepted that the pain of childbirth was inevitable because its cause and prevention were not studied. Modern scientific methods proved invaluable for the treatment of abnormal and unnatural cases, but the scientists took the easy path and, rather than seek a solution to the problem of pain, treated women in labor as if all were suffering from an illness or unnatural condition. For about fifty years, interference with straightforward cases has been the cause of more troubles for women and babies than anything else.

Now, happily, common sense has brought to light that childbirth is not an abnormal event or an illness, but an accomplishment which brings well-being and health to mothers and their babies and happiness to the home, and conscious birth a great benefit to the minds and bodies of both women and newborn infants.

Like everything else really worth possessing, we have to work for it and whatever good there may or may not be in a welfare state with a "free" national health service, a mother can't buy her babies with money nor can a husband be given his wife's children by local authorities. Men and women who are willing to learn their respective jobs for home- and family-making never regret the effort required. Babies either make or mar a home just as surely as the home will make or mar the child. The manner in which the children are born has a lot to do with the love and companionship of the mother and father as the years roll along.

That is why, after forty years of close association with homes and lives of young married people, I write with conviction, "Parents—pay attention to childbirth. It is the best investment for a happy, proud and successful life and it is available to poor and rich alike. It pays dividends more valuable than anything money can buy."

I do not promise every woman complete success, but 95 per cent of women can, with proper care, watch their babies born in full consciousness while having pain relief ready for immediate use if they want it. I do not promise "painless childbirth" and never have done so. Some women have their babies with no pain, but there is a certain amount of discomfort in most first labors, either backache or stretching feelings. If a mother and her attendants understand how to overcome these unpleasant sensations they become of so little consequence that only three or four women in a hundred wish for or need partial or total insensibility. It is no shame on a woman if she is not successful. We are not all made alike and success depends as much on the standard of teaching, care and treatment she gets as upon herself. However perfect her preparation, labor can be ruined by nurses and doctors who are indifferent to her efforts and don't help to carry out the teaching she has learned. Women must not blame themselves, or the method, if difficulty arises or if their attendants interfere without good reason.

I want to set out in this little book, shortly and quite simply, the bare necessities that every woman should know, without any elaborations or frills, in order to get the best result and yet spend the minimum amount of time in preparation. The housewife is a very busy person and we shouldn't ask her to do anything unless it is absolutely necessary. It is sometimes said by those who have never tried this method, "It is too simple to be true." I can only answer, "It is simple and it is true."

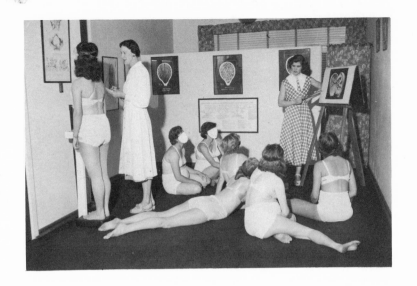

The Antenatal Class

FOR those who are teachers and instructors of women during pregnancy, I urge attention to the above illustration because it demonstrates the informality of classes. Do keep these classes friendly and informal, and give plenty of time for women to ask questions and to ventilate their problems. It is during these chats while patients are being weighed and shown some of the illustrations that they learn most and obtain confidence in the replies they are given. Secondly, do keep the classes small in order to maintain the personal touch. Eight or ten in a class is the maximum number that one instructress can handle adequately, and is ideal from the patient's point of view.

Education

WOMEN must be taught in ordinary, not medical, language how their babies are made and born and what they can do to make childbirth straightforward for themselves and their child. The five objectives of good midwifery are:

1. That women should be properly prepared during pregnancy and that they come into labor healthy, happy and confident.
2. That women should not be allowed to suffer unbearable discomfort in labor, whatever its cause.
3. That mothers and babies should be preserved in the best possible health during pregnancy, labor and delivery without injury to either the body or the mind. Two ways of causing greatest harm to the mind are to allow a woman to be terrified, and secondly, to allow a woman to endure prolonged, severe pain.
4. That every woman should have the opportunity of learning during pregnancy how pain in labor may be entirely avoided or diminished to such an extent that it becomes a willingly and easily borne discomfort.
5. That no woman should be left alone in labor.

Antenatal instruction, in order to obtain these ideals, has four main parts:

1. *Elementary Instruction* in the facts of pregnancy and childbirth that gives understanding and confidence and removes the fears and doubts that a woman may have planted in her mind by other people about bearing a baby.

2. Demonstration and practice of *Correct Breathing* so that the mother may be in good condition and the unborn baby well nourished as it grows in the womb. One of the lifelines of the baby is in the mother's breathing.

3. *Relaxation* and its application during pregnancy and labor.

4. *A few gentle exercises* to increase fitness for childbearing.

Of these four parts of instruction, education, as it is called, is first and foremost. This small book describes also breathing, relaxation and physical exercises and gives the reason why they help and how, and, combined with education, they make all the difference in the world to the mother and her baby when it is born. I say to mothers, "You will never regret preparing yourself properly for childbirth. It may take up a little time but every busy woman can find half an hour a day for a really important job."

By education, we mean being taught about pregnancy and childbirth. Some women say, "But it is natural, why should we know any more?" The answer is that in civilized countries there are still people who look upon childbirth as unnatural and this attitude often brings pain and injury to women and sometimes their babies as well. If we can avoid troubles which are avoidable and if we can make childbearing a happy event in a woman's life, why not do so? If a woman knows what goes on inside her when she is going to have a baby, she is more likely to take the advice of those who are looking after her. If she has a good reason for doing the right thing and knows how to do it, it is easier than being told to do something without knowing how or why.

Correct antenatal education tells in simple language how women can help themselves and accept the help their attendants are willing to give them; it does not take long to learn. In many towns, classes are organized for the instruction of expectant mothers, and the quality of the teaching is improving with experience. Trained women do much better in labor, and afterward with their babies, than those who are not taught.

If you are attending a clinic for breathing, relaxation and exercises you will probably have talks and ask questions while you are there. Many girls, before they leave school, are learning these days about animals having their young, how plants multiply and the way in which the human body takes nourishment from food and gets rid of waste, etc. When this opportunity has been given by sensible school-mistresses, it becomes much easier for the young woman to learn what goes on when she is pregnant and while the baby is being born.

But most women who start attending classes find childbirth a very interesting subject and want to know a good deal more about it. We advise them to get one of the books I have already mentioned because there is set out in detailed and easily understandable language just what "natural childbirth" in the widest sense means and how it can be achieved.

Now let me give you an outline of what you will be taught under the heading of education, and the reason for telling you is that you should have some idea of the wonderful provision that has been made for women to have babies. I hope that, like myself, you will also gain a tremendous respect for the genius of the Creator that such a remarkable series of events can be governed entirely beyond the power and even the understanding of man.

Fertilization

Nearly all animals, including human beings, have much the same principles of breeding. The female makes eggs and the male produces sperm. Eggs have to be fertilized by the sperm before they can grow into babies. Nature makes the process of fertilization attractive because the race must go on growing or it will die out. Women lay one egg every month (rarely two) about ten days after the menstruation or monthly period. The egg is shed by the small oval organ in which it is made, called the ovary, and travels down a fine tube. Here a sperm perforates its outer covering and so the egg becomes fertilized. After fertilization it continues on in the tube which leads to the womb or uterus, and when it arrives it grows onto and soon into the wall of the womb and the woman is known to be pregnant.

Menstruation

Each month a woman lays an egg just big enough to see without a magnifying glass and the uterus prepares its lining to make a good nest. If the egg is not fertilized, the lining of the uterus is thrown off and with it the wasted egg—that is the "show" of the monthly period. Each month an egg is laid and a new nest built until pregnancy occurs and then menstruation stops until some months after the baby is born.

The Womb

The virgin womb is a small muscular body about 2 × 1½ × 1 inches in length, breadth and depth. It is much the shape of a pear without a stalk. The stalk end fits down onto the top of the vagina and at the outlet of the vagina is the vulva. The lower end of the uterus is closed by a neck (or cervix) through which a small channel runs up into the main body of the organ.

Growth

The embryo—that is, the beginning of the baby—grows very fast. At four weeks it is a sixth of an inch long and at eight weeks it is one and a quarter inches long, and at sixteen weeks it is seven inches long. By twenty weeks the baby is completely formed, and many born at twenty-eight weeks have survived and done well. The full term is forty weeks or nine calendar months. The average weight is about seven pounds and the length, nineteen to twenty inches. During its growing life, the baby has been protected by a "bag of waters" in which it lives. By being in this bag of waters, or liquor as it is called, it doesn't get injured from any direct violence and also it is kept at a constant temperature by the mother, so she can move about and do all sorts of things without upsetting the baby or the little house in which it is living.

The growth of the baby inside the womb is maintained through the mother's blood. There is a wonderful organ known as the placenta which develops with the baby, and is able to filter from the large blood vessels of the womb the food required by the baby. It knows what the baby wants and takes it and passes it on by a cord to the infant's navel, and through the cord the waste and unwanted material are returned to be disposed of by the mother. So it becomes clear we can help to have *healthy babies by eating and drinking the right things.*

One of the most important foods is oxygen. Adults cannot live a quarter of an hour without it, and we breathe it in through our lungs. The baby doesn't use its lungs but takes its oxygen from the placenta straight into its bloodstream; therefore, by correct breathing, the mother can supply as much oxygen to the baby as it requires, and it is surprising to learn that not one woman in fifty breathes properly. That is why we teach how to improve *breathing during pregnancy*—the baby as well as the mother benefits.

Full Term

Toward the end of pregnancy the uterus is large and fills the abdomen almost up to the level of the ribs. The womb, the placenta, the bag of waters and the baby may weigh twelve pounds or more, and this extra weight and altered shape must be carried well or women may have backaches, headaches or bad digestion. Most women with faulty posture and poor carriage at mid-pregnancy breathe badly and feel miserable. So we teach a woman how to carry herself well in spite of her altered weight and shape. No woman need lose a good figure because she bears a baby. With proper care and a little effort, she can be more attractive after than before pregnancy, especially to her husband, which creates mutual admiration and affection as well as both physical and mental unity.

Labor—the Expected Date

Many women are very hazy about the day when the baby is due to arrive. Let me give you a short note on that. When a baby is ready it will come, and we should be prepared for it to arrive from 14 days before the calculated date up to 14 days after. That is quite within the range of a normal, healthy baby's time. Pregnancy is, on the average, 280 days, counting from the first day of the last monthly period. The simplest way is to go back three months and add seven days. For instance, the first day of the last monthly period on November 5—back October 5—September 5—August 5 —add seven days and you come to August 12.

The Onset of Labor

The baby gives warning of the onset of labor in three ways:
1. Rhythmical contractions of the womb coming on regularly but gradually more frequent.
2. Leaking from the bag of waters, a nearly odorless and clear liquid which cannot be controlled.
3. A show (bloodstained) mixed with heavy mucus.
Any one or more than one of these is a signal to call the midwife

or doctor, or go to the maternity hospital, according to the arrangements you have made for the birth of your baby. Labor for first babies is slow, and strong, healthy women should expect anything from ten to sixteen hours, or even longer. Some are fortunate in having their babies more quickly, but others have to go as long as twenty-four hours; however, time is not an important factor to a properly instructed woman.

Labor is divided into three stages: *

The First Stage is taken up by the opening of the womb to let the baby out into the vagina, which becomes the lower part of the birth canal.

The Second Stage, which may last from one-half to two hours, is the passage of the baby from the uterus, after it has fully opened, through the birth canal and out of the body.

The Third Stage is the expulsion of the afterbirth (which is the placenta).

This is the normal series of events in a healthy birth and naturally should not be painful. The first stage requires patience and self control, very difficult for some; there is hard work in the second or pushing stage; but no other natural function is painful, why should there be unbearable pain in childbirth?

The Cause of Pain in Normal Labor

If I explain simply the cause of pain in normal labor, the reason for preparation for childbirth will be clear to you.

The womb has three layers of muscle:

a. One going up the back, over the top and down the front; these muscle bands are mainly in the middle and upper part of the womb. (Fig. 1.)

b. The middle layer is a mass of twisted and tortuous muscles in which the big blood vessels lie. (Fig. 2.)

* Full information on labor may be found in *Childbirth Without Fear.*

MUSCLES OF THE UTERUS

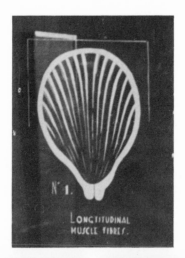

Nº 1.

LONGITUDINAL
MUSCLE FIBRES.

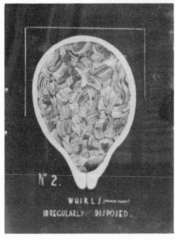

Nº 2.

WHIRLS (muscle fibres)
IRREGULARLY DISPOSED.

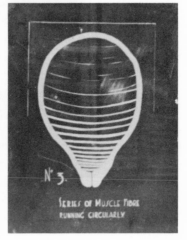

Nº 3.

SERIES OF MUSCLE FIBRE
RUNNING CIRCULARLY

c. The inner layer goes round the womb in a circular manner and it is almost entirely in the lower part of the womb. (Fig. 3.) (See diagrams.)

So the outer muscle by contraction presses the baby down, through and ultimately out of the uterus. The middle muscles by contracting squeeze the blood out of the walls of the uterus and when they relax the blood vessels fill up again. The inner muscles by contracting maintain the shape of the uterus and also close the outlet. These circular muscles should be loose and relaxed when the long muscles contract and gradually open the womb to push the baby out. Unfortunately they contract and become tight if a woman is frightened by labor or during labor, with the result that the muscles that empty and the muscles that close the uterus work against each other. When you have two big groups of muscles working against each other, they soon begin to hurt and in a short time the pain becomes very severe. We speak of this as the Fear-Tension-Pain Syndrome of childbirth, for a woman who is afraid unconsciously resists the birth of her baby and increases the tension within the uterus. The absence of give-and-take of the muscles causes nearly all the pains and distresses of labor.

I am not, of course, referring to the few women who have something wrong inside, but to normal women with healthy babies and a good birth canal, and that means at least ninety-five women in a hundred. So, if a woman's fear of labor is removed by understanding, what happens? The muscles that close the womb before labor will be loose and easily stretched when the muscles that empty the womb start to expel the baby. The tension caused by resistance will not be there to make pain, and that is why every mother should be taught the truth about childbirth and why education is the most important part of preparation. The best way of avoiding unnecessary pain is to understand what occurs during labor and how to meet the changes.

Fear-Tension-Pain

This fear-tension-pain series of events is experienced by every-body in circumstances very similar in some ways. The bowel is full, the desire to empty is acute, it pushes against our active restraint but the time and place are not convenient. We are afraid to stop resisting, it is uncomfortable and becomes painful. And again, we have a strong urge to pass water, the bladder is full but the right place is not available. We dare not relax the muscles that close the bladder, we are afraid of the social and domestic repercussions so we suffer an increasing pain, sometimes an agony, until resistance is removed and the comfort is experienced of relaxing the outlet and emptying the distended, contracting organ.

It is just this same principle in labor. Fear of pain causes resist-ance to the massive muscles of the womb and so tension and pain. Fear of disaster causes resistance to the less powerful muscles of the bowel and bladder but how painful it may become after a time. So, by removing fear through understanding, relaxation is possible and that is why we teach how it is done.

A relaxed woman allows the "door" or outlet of the womb to open easily. A tense woman is closing the door against her baby. During labor, the big muscle of the uterus is working, and when big muscles are used they require more fuel, just as a car to go faster or pull harder must have more petrol. We don't feel our muscles working if we are fit, but we do breathe faster and deeper and that is how we get extra fuel. During labor, breathing is im-portant to both the mother and the baby; that is why special atten-tion is given in this book to breathing and relaxation, and women who practice these two simple parts of preparation not only help themselves by avoiding discomforts but they keep fit during the hours of hard work and do not tire so easily.

One of the biggest differences between those who have worked to be prepared well for labor and the woman who has not done so is that they will keep the uterus strong until its job is over and remain strong themselves, not suffering the exhaustion that we see in so many uninstructed women. Equally important is the effect upon the baby. There is plenty of fuel to see it through the birth canal and into the world to greet its mother with a powerful yell immediately it is born.

The Correlation Chart

THE correlation chart shows the course of the large majority of natural labors. Midwives and teachers will see these changes and by recognizing them be able to give the kind of support needed by women through the different phases of labor. Women who study this sequence of events learn what to expect and how to act and behave as the changes of sensation and mental attitude arise. No two labors are quite alike but many women have checked up these changes for me during labor and the general opinion is that this chart shows the important incidents. Some women experience all of them and others some but not all. It will be a great help to study it carefully.

CORRELATION OF THE PHYSICAL ANI

Onset of Labor	"A"	Approximate Duration	"B"
1. Rhythmic Contractions	INITIATION	PRIMIP.*	TRANSITION
2. Leaking of the Waters	Expectancy	3–12 hrs.	"Pain Period of Labor
3. The Show		MULTIP.†	when pain occurs
		2–6 hrs.	
ANTENATAL PREPARATION		CONTRACTIONS	4/5th DILATATION OF
ANTICIPATION OF LABOR		DEFINITE RHYTHM	CERVIX OF UTERUS
		Shortening Interval	

FIRST STAGE OF LABOR

Patience, confidence and self-control; nothing to be afraid of.
Relaxation DURING contractions.
- A. 1. Commencement—exhilaration and animation.
  2. Uterine cervix dilates 1/5th–2/5ths. Cheerfulness maintained.
  3. Uterine cervix 2/5ths to 3/5ths. Taking labor more seriously. Desire for compan ionship. Relax throughout contractions.
  4. Cervix dilated 3/5ths–4/5ths. Strengthening contractions introduce conflict. Cor fidence versus fear, relaxation versus tension. The FIRST TEST of self-control an faith.
  5. Uterine cervix 4/5ths to full dilatation. Acute sensitiveness to words and noise Horror of being left alone in labor. Backache in 80 per cent of women. Demand fo understanding companionship. The SECOND TEST of self-control and faith. Relaxa tion becomes difficult with the change of breathing required for expulsive contrac tions.

SECOND STAGE OF LABOR

Concentrated hard work associated with uterine activity. Later drowsiness of mind and bod during relaxation now BETWEEN expulsive contractions.
- B. 6. Expulsive reflex not strong. Temporary revival of personality and determinatio Backache ceases. No discomfort but hard work.
  7. Onset of drowsiness as head progresses down birth canal. Expulsive effort stronge
  8. Head in pelvic cavity. Woman's true self evident. Sometimes discretion and di crimination "low."

* Primip. means a woman having her first baby.
† Multip. means a woman who has already had one or more babies.

MOTIONAL PHENOMENA OF LABOR

APPROXIMATE DURATION PRIMIP. ½– 2 hrs. MULTIP. 5 mins.–½ hr.	"C" TRANSFIGURATION Delight & Pride	APPROXIMATE DURATION PRIMIP. AND MULTIP. 2 mins. to 35 mins. sometimes longer	RESTITUTION and Refreshment
WELL-ESTABLISHED EXPULSIVE REFLEX	BIRTH OF BABY'S HEAD	INFANT IN MOTHER'S ARMS	A state of peaceful happiness and pride of achievement in which Stage C is indelibly imprinted on the mind. Childbirth has become a wonderful experience not to be feared but gratefully to be remembered for all time.

SECOND STAGE OF LABOR (continued)

9. Head reaches pelvic floor. Sudden impatience and desire to escape; often careless of words and appearance. THIRD TEST of self-control.
10. Stretching and thinning of perineum. Exasperation threatens perseverance and patience.
11. Before head dilates outlet of birth canal. Attendant induces quiet patience and confidence.
12. Stretching of vulva and crowning. Discretion very weak. The burning feeling round vulva threatens control. The FOURTH TEST of self-control and faith in attendants.
13. Birth of the head. Drowsiness replaced by mental alertness.
14. Dramatic change of interest from herself to the newborn baby.

THIRD STAGE OF LABOR

15. Sound of the first cry. Incredulity: all weariness vanishes.
16. Sight and touch of her infant. Fascinated wonder, enchantment.
17. Her infant in her arms. State of emotional ecstasy which varies in character and intensity in different women.
18. Strong and prolonged contraction of uterus. A reflex advantage of co-operation and consciousness.
19. Rapid expulsion of placenta in vagina. Painless miniature second-stage type of contractions.
20. Complete expulsion of placenta with minimum blood loss. Satisfied sense of achievement. Happiness and pride. No exhaustion and no shock.
21. A hot drink of tea with plenty of sugar. The baby returned to her arms for warmth, cuddling and baby talk. The husband returns to join in the welcome.

Respiration

No ONE can work to the best of her ability either physically or mentally if she does not breathe correctly. It is *the* bad habit that causes more illness than any other.

During pregnancy it is of the utmost importance that as much fresh air as possible is taken into the lungs with the least effort. It is required by the mother and her growing child. Correct breathing during labor not only helps the womb to expel the baby, but keeps the baby strong and in good condition while it is being born. The secret is the control of respiration—that is, breathing in and out. I repeat this because it is important.

Fresh air is taken into the lungs, while are like a very fine sponge made of minute air spaces and even smaller blood vessels. The walls are so thin that the oxygen from the air passes into the blood and the waste gas from the blood passes into the air space, so by breathing we take in pure gas and get rid of "fumes."

Most people use rather less than four-fifths of their air space, so to keep up supplies they have to breathe five times for every four breaths of a good breather. This means more work for the muscles concerned with breathing and more work for the heart to pump the blood around the body. In pregnancy that can become a strain and even a discomfort for a woman.

First learn to *breathe deeply*. To do this, let your tummy go loose, open your mouth and fill up your chest as full as you can, then let the air out. Lean slightly forward and force out the last possible breath. You won't do any harm so don't be afraid to take deep in-and-out breaths. Do this slowly, putting your hands flat on

way for a minute or two before repeating the exercise. It is well to repeat this two or three times; then you will grasp the idea quickly. The final results will give you a beautiful sensation, a feeling of complete relaxation, quiet in mind and body, and in this condition you should continue for twenty to thirty minutes.

A good tip to remember is that, particularly at this time, the mind tends to roam, so keep it under control by concentrating on the job of relaxing.

Don't expect to be perfect right away. Sometimes it takes a lot of practice, for few people are what we can term "natural relaxers," but perseverance is worth while and can apply to everyone. Don't be worried if you go to sleep—many women do—for we live lives of considerable stress and there is more physical weariness than is usually recognized. Relaxation is not only for pregnancy and labor, but if it is continued it lays a foundation of good health afterward as a means of escape from unnecessary worry. Women who practice relaxation enhance their natural beauty; the posture and carriage of the body become attractive and they lose self-consciousness or awkwardness in their association with both friends and strangers.

Remember, it is the state of tension that undermines both health and happiness in the rush and scurry of modern living. Time spent to overcome mental and physical tension not only aids a woman to an easier and happy birth, but to a healthier and more efficient way of life as a mother, a wife and a member of the community.

RELAXATION NEAR FULL TERM

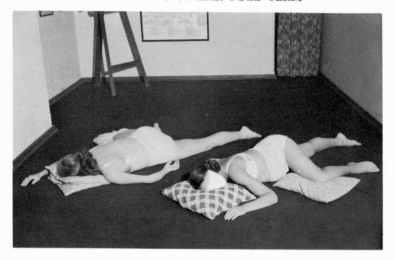

LATERAL POSITION

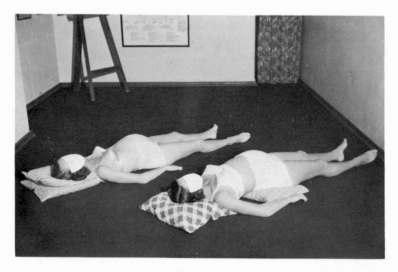

ON BACK

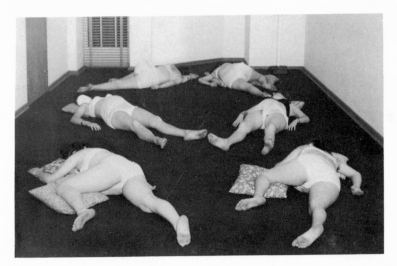

CLASS PRACTICING RELAXATION

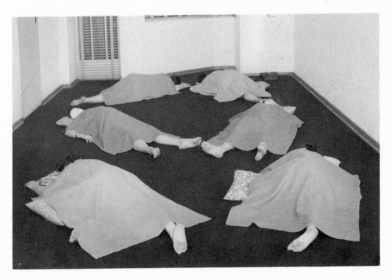

CLASS RESTS AFTER PRACTICING RELAXATION

Positions for Labor

THE position for relaxing when the *first* stage of labor is established must be practiced. In plate 2 (p. 30) the woman is shown relaxing on her left side. She may, from time to time, change to the right side or, if it is comfortable, on her back for a short while, but the position illustrated proves to be the best for free respiration and complete relaxation during first-stage contractions.

Don't hang the arm over the sharp edge of a bed or sofa; put a pad under it, or bring the end of the pillow down so that it rests on the soft support.

Plate 1 on page 31 illustrates the position during the *second* stage of labor. For many years, women in the British Isles have been delivered on the left side, with the buttock on or over the edge of the bed. It is argued that when the midwife is alone it gives her better control of the patient. This is all wrong and those who were trained that way should change.

The position in this picture has many advantages over any other. It is the attitude of squatting with the weight on the lower back instead of on the feet. This enables the woman and her attendant to work in full view of each other and if the patient's right foot is placed on the hip of the midwife, she can hold the left leg up and press the knees widely open herself. The size of the pelvic outlet is at its biggest and the muscles required to press down are free to work their hardest when squatting.

The woman can see her baby born and the midwife can deliver the infant in the correct manner to prevent injury at the outlet. As soon as a contraction passes, the legs are rested as in plates 2 and 3 (pp. 31, 32) and the blanket drawn over the mother.

The back is resting on a bedrest or a number of pillows to bring it to an angle of forty-five degrees to the labor bed and a small pillow is put under the head to keep it slightly forward when relaxing. This labor position makes the whole process easier and less exhausting for both the patient and the attendant.

FIRST STAGE OF LABOR

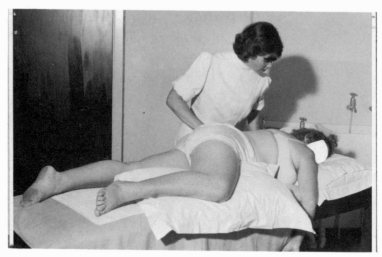

1. Patient in Relaxed Position with Attendant Rubbing Back

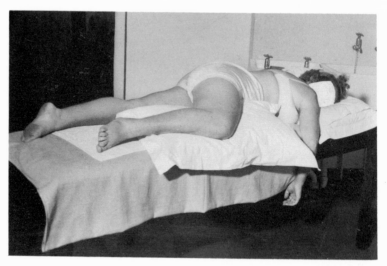

2. Patient Relaxing to Contraction in Advanced First Stage

SECOND STAGE OF LABOR

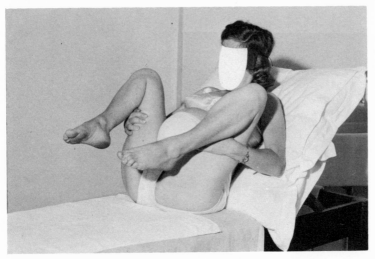

1. PATIENT IN POSITION FOR BEARING-DOWN EFFORT

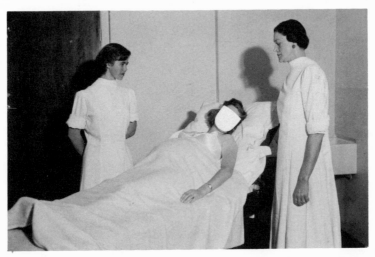

2. PATIENT RELAXED BETWEEN CONTRACTIONS WITH ATTENDANT ON
EITHER SIDE

SECOND STAGE OF LABOR (continued)

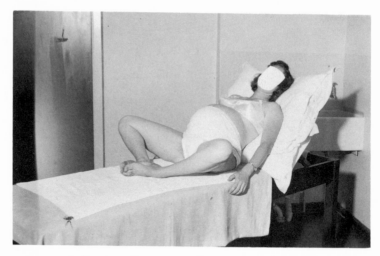

3. PATIENT RELAXED AT PERIOD OF CROWNING

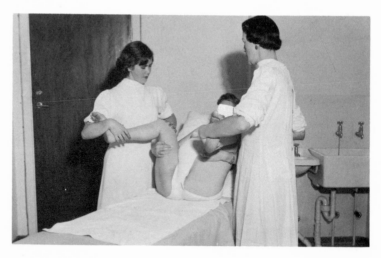

4. PATIENT IN POSITION FOR EXPULSIVE EFFORT WITH ATTENDANTS
HOLDING LIMBS

Exercises

You will find it very much easier to do these exercises by examining the pictures and reading the instructions underneath them.

Just one or two words of advice.

Never do your exercises quickly, and do think what you are doing the whole time.

Concentrate on the regularity of your breathing in conjunction with the movements described.

Don't do any exercising with your arms above your head. Shoulder height is the maximum to which you ever bring your arms during antenatal exercises.

Remember that those for stretching the adductor muscles as in Figs. 1B and 1C, Exercise 2, are most important because they not only help to make the pelvic outlet larger when the legs are in that position during the second stage of labor, but they also make it very much easier for you to push down when the baby needs your help. You can see your attendant's face and understand his or her advice more clearly, and *you can see your baby born.*

In Exercise 4, in position 1A, take a deep breath in and then let it out again while adopting position 1C. Having returned to position 1A you can take a very deep breath in and on adopting position 1B you breathe out again before you return to the normal, which is position 1A.

Exercise 5 is fully explained underneath the pictures, as are all the other illustrations.

Don't exaggerate the importance of exercises. They make you feel fit and help both correct breathing and relaxation, and that makes them valuable, but a woman with a well-trained mind unable to do any exercises has her baby much more easily than the highly trained athletic body of a woman who knows little or nothing of childbirth. We are not preparing you for an athletic event, but for a natural, common-sense experience in which a certain degree of physical fitness has advantages.

CHART OF EXERCISES

Exercise No. 1
This is a respiratory exercise.

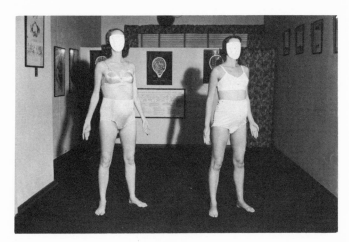

Fig. 1A

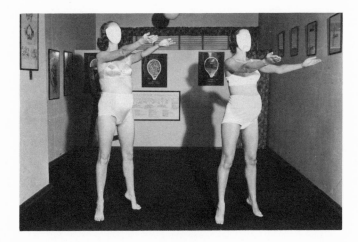

Fig. 1B

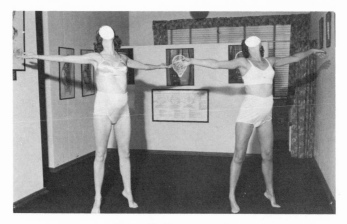

Fig. 1C (Exercise 1)

Stand with the feet comfortably apart, the hands at the sides, palms to the front. Raise the hands in front of the body to shoulder level, at the same time rising on the toes. Swing the arms outward, throwing the head slightly backward. Complete this movement during deep inspiration, slowly resuming starting position with expiration. Repeat six times.

Exercise No. 2

For loosening the knees and hip joints, toning up the muscles of the legs and feet and stretching the adductor or riding muscles on the inside of the thigh.

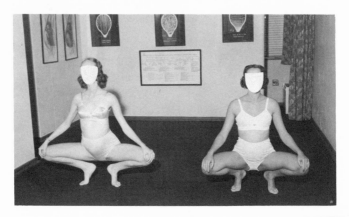

Fig. 1A

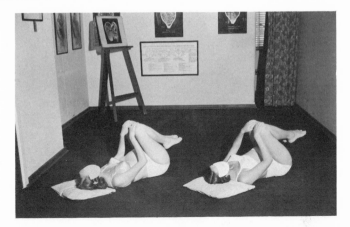

FIG. 1B (EXERCISE 2)

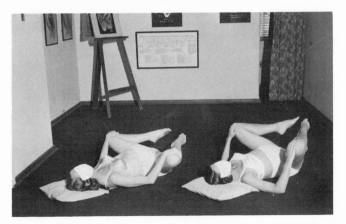

FIG. 1C (EXERCISE 2)

This exercise is to facilitate the best position for delivery of the child, for in this position as shown in Fig. 4 (p. 32) the pelvic diameter is enlarged. Breathe in and rise on the toes, sink down to the position of squatting or sitting on the heels. Place the hands on the knees and stretch the legs wide open, keeping the back upright. Rise to standing position, dropping the heels. If the balance cannot be retained at first, with one hand hold on to a support. Repeat five times.

Adductor stretching is very important. This exercise can also be done while lying on the back with the knees flexed, allowing them to fall outward and the hands to press them widely apart (Figs. 1B and 1C).

EXERCISE NO. 3

This loosens and mobilizes the lower spine and pelvic joints. Prevents and sometimes relieves backache.

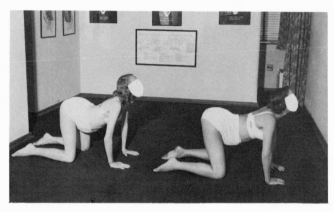

FIG. 1A

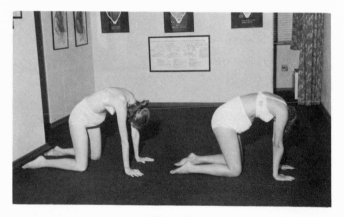

FIG. 1B

Assume position (Fig. 1A), the hands about shoulder-width apart, the knees approximately 8 inches apart, the back hollow, elbows slightly bent and head well back. In this position take deep breath. Tuck the head between the arms, raise the back, at the same time straightening the arms, and pull the buttocks inward, allowing the breath to be expelled as the back arches (Fig. 1B). Resume position (Fig. 1A) and do this six times, slowly and firmly.

EXERCISE No. 4

This not only loosens and mobilizes the pelvic joints, and the articulation of the spine, but facilitates a free and controlled deep-breathing exercise.

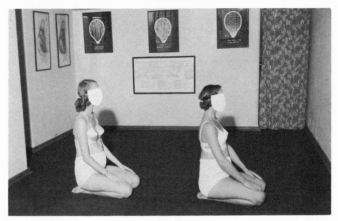

FIG. 1A

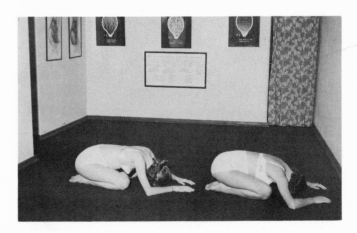

FIG. 1B

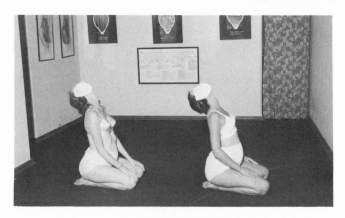

FIG. 1C (EXERCISE 4)

Kneel as in position (Fig. 1A) on the heels with the hands on the knees, which are fully flexed and about a foot apart. With the back straight take a deep breath in, bend forward, breathing out until the elbows and arms are flat upon the floor in front of the knees (Fig. 1B). Breathe in as the body is raised to the original position and complete the movement by pressing on the knees with hands, hollowing the back and lifting the chin (Fig. 1C). Return to normal position and breathing. Pause and repeat eight times.

EXERCISE No. 5

For strengthening muscles of abdomen and thighs.

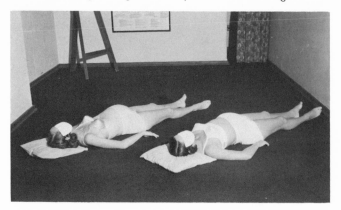

FIG. 1A

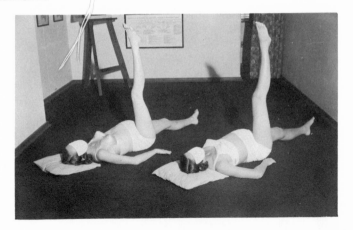

FIG. 1B (EXERCISE 5)

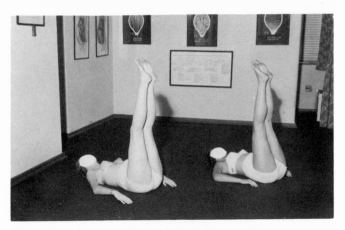

FIG. 1C (EXERCISE 5)

Lie on the back. While breathing in raise right leg, without bending the knee, as high as it will go comfortably. Lower it slowly to the floor during exhalation. Do the same with the left leg, and repeat alternately six times each.

Raise both legs together (Fig. 1C), bending the feet up rather than pointing the toes. Lower legs slowly to the floor. Legs up, breathe in—legs down, breathe out. This may be difficult at first but with practice it will become easier and performed without strain. It is an excellent exercise for pregnant women. The intervals between the repetitions should be longer than in less strenuous movements.

EXERCISE NO. 6

For tensing and relaxing the muscles of the front of the chest. This exercise increases the circulation of the tissue under the breasts and appears to enhance the establishment of adequate lactation. It differs from the others in that it is also used for training in holding the breath.

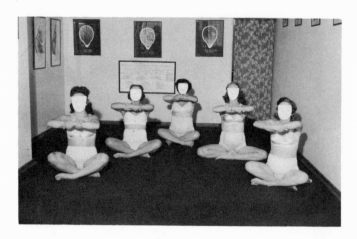

Grip firmly behind the wrists. Push the skin up the forearm, thereby tensing the arms and the muscles of the chest. Relax and repeat. The breath is held in inspiration while this is done ten times, taking about ten seconds. This time is gradually increased until the breath can be held comfortably for twenty seconds, which is of considerable aid in the expulsive stage of labor when a contraction may last for ten to sixteen seconds without a remission allowing expiration to take place.

The Hygiene of Pregnancy

Preparation and Care of the Breasts

There are one or two points about personal hygiene, that is to say looking after yourself during pregnancy, and first of all perhaps the most important is the preparation of the breasts for feeding the baby.

On the whole, this has been made far too much of in recent years and there is very little doubt that *properly supported breasts* need very little care. They must be kept in the right position and the nipples kept clean with warm water. Great care should be taken that the breast is not handled roughly or violently rubbed and massaged, advice which one occasionally hears.

During the last ten or twelve weeks there may be a few drops of a very thick, yellow secretion from the breasts and warm water will undoubtedly soften that. Very gentle pressure at the base of the nipple with the thumb and forefinger will clear the little openings into the breast in case this substance, called colostrum, gets too thick, but it should, I repeat, be done extremely gently and without any force at all.

If the nipple is slightly retracted and doesn't stand out as it should after warm bathing, then it is best to take the advice of the doctor at the antenatal clinic as to whether or no he suggests the wearing of a shield * which tends to make the nipple stand out more and enable the baby to feed with comfort and ease.

I remember in the old days as a student we were told to put

* For many years I have found Waller's breast shield efficient.

43

"Friar's balsam" around the nipples, but that is undoubtedly a very bad thing to do. There should be no application whatever, and the softer and more elastic the nipple can be kept so much the better for the woman who wishes to feed her baby as, indeed, the large majority of women do. I can only repeat, there should never be any pressure on the breast or the nipple of the pregnant woman and that not only refers to the type of brassière worn but the manner of keeping the breast clean and preparing it for lactation.

The Skin

You must take care of the skin of the body. Very frequently in pregnancy women develop areas of brown pigment which give them a good deal of worry, but it all goes after pregnancy and as long as you keep your skin clean and soft with a good alkaline soap or one of the many creams that can be bought to prevent cracking, it is well worth while and you are not troubled with spots and unnecessary discomforts of the face, hands and arms, etc.

The Hair

This also applies to the hair. During pregnancy sometimes there is a tendency for the hair to fall out or become rather lifeless and displeasing. I still prefer just a few drops of the very old-fashioned oil of macassar. It was used by my grandmothers, and my patients have used it during the last ten years and find it very advantageous. Just give the hair a good brushing and rub a few drops of macassar oil into the scalp and see that the scalp moves freely on your skull. The chances are, if you wash it once a week as you should, you will have no trouble at all—it will keep its life and look better after pregnancy than before.

Wearing Apparel

THE following plates show the Grantly Dick-Read maternity belt, the Grantly Dick-Read maternity and nursing brassière and two kinds of stocking supporters:

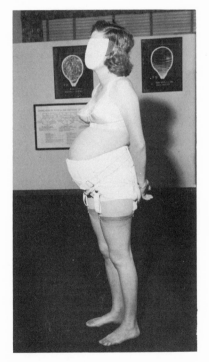

GRANTLY DICK-READ MATERNITY BELT

The Grantly Dick-Read maternity belt and brassière are obtainable from Treasure Cot Ltd., 103 Oxford Street, London, W.1.

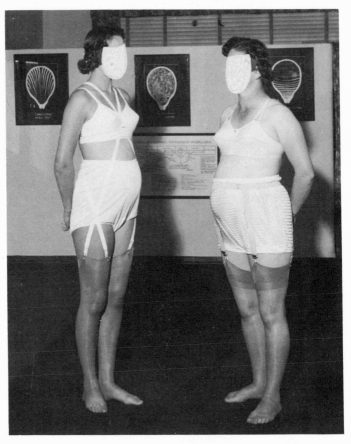

STOCKING SUPPORTERS

The shoulder stocking support on the left of the plate is taken from the Lane Bryant maternity catalogue, U.S.A.

1   2

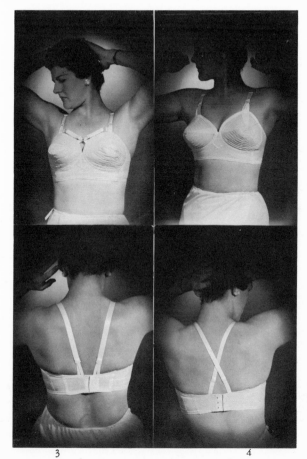

3   4

THE GRANTLY DICK-READ BRASSIÈRES

1. Maternity Brassière—with release fasteners for each cup for feeding, cross
   straps to adjust before and after feeding and inner pocket for absorbent pad.
2. All-Purpose Brassière—with adjustable and detachable straps for crossing,
   designed to prompt good posture, free respiration and firm support.
3. Straight straps—Back view. Lower band fastened on first hooks.
4. Cross straps—Back view. Lower band fastened on second hooks.

(Plates 3 and 4 refer to both 1 and 2.)

Appendix

A Simple Guide to the Planning of an Antenatal School of Instruction on the Grantly Dick-Read Principles

The Purpose of the Antenatal School is to offer to women the opportunity of having their babies naturally with the minimum of discomfort and unnecessary interference in attaining the most glorious of woman's achievements.

Teaching must be simple and understandable to all types of women, covering the four essentials:

1. EDUCATION (*see* p. 6)
2. CORRECT BREATHING
3. RELAXATION
4. EXERCISES concurrent with breathing

Included in the teaching is simple anatomy, the functioning of the womb and its muscles, personal hygiene, care of the breasts and skin, proper support of the breasts and abdomen (where necessary), care of the hair, teeth, fingernails, feet and clothing, diet and mothercraft, and the principles of postnatal care.

Instructresses must have a knowledge of the subject and an ability to teach. Women who have had their babies naturally are often excellent teachers; nurses and physiotherapists must be trained in the natural childbirth procedures to obtain good results. Classes should be conducted in a friendly way without regimentation or a display of authority but with quiet companionship. Keen concentration on the work gives women the confidence to ask questions and do their best to become efficient.

Pattern and Structure of the School. Three rooms are required, one for teaching, one as a changing room (divided into cubicles to allow for two persons to a cubicle) with a washbasin and toilet, and a small anteroom for secretarial and office work. In the main room, the floor should be covered with soft rubberized or similar material, and an accurate weighing machine should be kept in this room for weight checks at each attendance. For other equipment allow one mat, one small blanket and two small pillows per pupil (the pillows with removable covers allowing for easy washing), with the following diagrams: *

* Dickinson-Belskie Birth Atlas and Eva Schuchardt diagrams are available from the Maternity Center Association, 48 East 92nd Street, New York 28, N.Y.
The Grantly Dick-Read Correlation Chart and diagrams of the uterus and the

The Dickinson Birth Atlas and the Eva Schuchardt diagrams.

The Grantly Dick-Read Correlation Chart and diagrams of uterus.

Photographs from *Childbirth Without Fear* and/or illustrations from *Introduction to Motherhood*.

CLASSES. Ten classes in a course including two lectures on labor which husbands are encouraged to attend and which take place between the 32nd and 36th weeks. Classes commence at 18 to 20 weeks' pregnancy, eight pupils at a time, but not more than ten for one instructress. They should be within four to six weeks of the same period of gestation so far as possible, and experience has shown that it is preferable and makes a happier class altogether if the multiparæ and primiparæ are not segregated. Pupils attend once in two weeks and the class lasts approximately one to one and a half hours, and progressively covers the teaching set out above.

In this way, under the organization of two instructresses, an antenatal school can be efficiently run maintaining four classes a day, or three during the day and one in the early evening so that women who work during the day may attend after office hours, i.e.,

9:30 A.M. to 11 A.M., 11:30 A.M. to 1 P.M., 2:30 P.M. to 4 P.M. and 4:30 P.M. to 6 P.M or 6 P.M. to 7:30 P.M.

The lectures can also be held in the evening if this is more convenient.

It is understood that routine clinical examination will be carried out by the doctor in charge of the case or the staff at the hospital which the patient attends. Women should be encouraged to attend the classes, where strict records of weight (each class) and other relevant data are kept so that any important observations may be communicated to the doctor in charge without delay. This has frequently proved to be of great value to women and those concerned with them.

Extra-curricular arrangements can be made for the classes to hear the phonograph recording of a natural childbirth or see the 16 mm. sound and color film of three natural births entitled *Childbirth Without Fear*.

---

photographs from *Childbirth Without Fear* or illustrations from *Introduction to Motherhood* are found in these Dick-Read books, all published by Harper & Brothers, 49 East 33rd Street, New York 16, N.Y.

An LP record, *Natural Childbirth,* is available at your local record store, or from the Westminster Recording Company, Inc., 275 Seventh Ave., New York 1, N.Y.

The film *Childbirth Without Fear* is available for rent or purchase from the United World Films, Inc., 1445 Park Ave., New York 29, N.Y.

Index

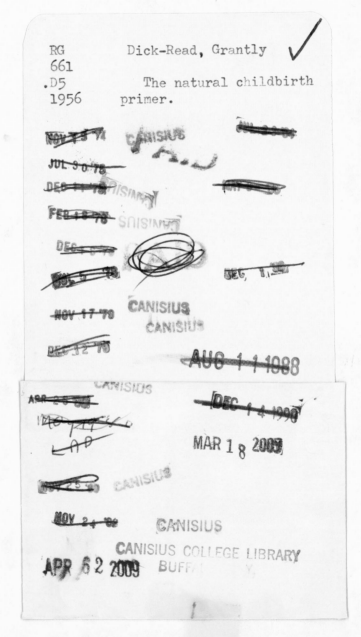